If I Told You…
Would You Listen?

By Cheryl Matthynssens
Cancer Fighter and Survivor

Copyright © 2019 by Cheryl Matthynssens

All rights reserved. No part of this publication may be reproduced, distributed or transmitted in any form or by any means, without prior written permission.

ISBN: 9781793128829

If I Told You, Would You Listen?

If I told you would you listen?
If our eyes met would you turn and walk away?
Would you pretend you didn't hear me?
Would you forget that we were friends until that day?

If I told you would you listen?
I just pretend to be so strong.
I can't really be the center, the pillar,
the one you counted on.

You ask me how to help?
Do you really want to know?
Is this politeness I am seeing?
Is your offer just for show?

I need my son to take my place,
My daughter to take his hand.
They have to help the others,
For I no longer can.

Don't tell me what you learned from me,
Show me how in what you do.
Don't tell me I can beat this,
Only God knows my time is through.

Don't tell me that I got this,
Even the oak tree bows low
The parasite seeks its roots
Though the tree will never show.

If I told you would you listen?

I am scared each and every day.
I hurt almost every minute
These words are what I'd say.

I am not afraid to die,
my life has been well lived
I have no yearning dreams to miss
My goals are now short-lived.

Yet fear you ask, you said its daily show?
If dying doesn't scare you then what fear plagues you so?
I fear the addict not yet saved, the lessons not yet taught,
I fear the pain of family when last my breath is naught.

If I told you would you listen?
There is nothing here to fear?
Each day is precious and fulfilled
And days turn into years.

If I told you, would you listen?
What would I have you do?
Sit down and make this list
Every day for it pursue.

1. Get up each morning with a list of things your grateful
for, read it through and fully before you leave your door.
2. When people talk then listen, don't think just what to
say. It will make you smart and interesting, as you go your
separate way.
3. Pay forward every kindness, even just a smile. These
vibes they are important, it only takes a while.
4. Live your day its fullest, don't linger through its
flight. Is it needed? Is it just? Is it doing what is right?

5. Before your day has ended, lay out your plan tomorrow. Say forgiveness where it's needed, let go of every
sorrow.

I told you did you listen?
Or will you heart the words away.
Will it bring a tear but not a change?
Do you now know what to say?

If you do those tasks with open heart and mind,
you need not fear my loss for I will walk your every mile.
My memory will live in every deed, immortal for all
time,
For every kindness given, I live for just awhile.

I told you... did you listen?

Introduction

Hello!

My name is Cheryl Lynn Matthynssens. If you have picked up this book, it is likely that you or someone you know has been diagnosed with cancer or some other life-threatening illness. I am so glad you picked this up. For future reference, I will be using the word cancer a lot as this is MY illness. Feel free to substitute any other life threatening or debilitating illness. I think my words will apply even if your illness is not cancer.

I will be telling my whole story near the end of this book, but I wanted to give a short introduction, so you know my experience and expertise. I am fifty-three years old. I have stage four colon cancer that has metastasized multiple times and is now in my liver and lungs. I have been fighting for over four years.

I felt qualified to write this short book not only because I am a cancer fighter, but also because I am a counselor and life coach. I will not be relying on my knowledge alone. I am in touch with other survivors and will share some things by other experts. The names of the survivors will not be shared for their personal privacy.

The most important thing I want to share right now is that if you have been diagnosed with cancer or another life-threatening disease you are NOT ALONE! As the fighter, we are only as alone as we decide to be. I will be sure to share ways to gain a support system around you.

The second thing I want you to know is that I will not be sugar coating and carefully crafting a polite way to share information. I will be speaking plainly, fighter to fighter, or fighter to support system member. Every time someone has tried to talk around the issue, it has been up-setting. I will not do that to you.

This book is not designed to be read in order. Go to the sections that are most applicable to your role in the battle to come. That all being said, let's get started.

You have Cancer

"You have cancer."

Those words are etched into every fiber of my being. Where I was. Whose voice it was. How it was said. Those three little words can change a life forever. For some it is a sign to put one's affairs in order, to others it is a warning, and to a third group it is signal for one of the hardest fights they will ever experience.

I want to tell you this! You do not have to let cancer change who you are unless you want it to. For some, it is a wakeup call and a serious look back on what they have been doing. I know for me, I realized that I was not being the person I would want others to remember. If you like who you are and where you have been, don't let cancer define you. Trust me, that is easier said than done.

One of the hardest parts for those fighting that do not have a terminal diagnosis is to keep moving forward. It is easy to convince ourselves that since a doctor told us we are sick, we now must act sick. What is worse, others treat us as if we are about to die even if the diagnosis is long term but not terminal. If you are terminal, I have a chapter just for you.

You tell someone you have cancer and you hear "I am so sorry!" I hate those words. I often want to scream… "What are you sorry about?" I know though, it is because they don't know what else to say. In society, people equate the word cancer with death, but a lot of people find remission or live for many years following the diagnosis today. When you say I have cancer what they hear is 'I am going to die.' Keep in mind that new treatments are coming out all the time.

"I am so sorry." The reason I hate it is that it is hard not to feel sorry for yourself when everyone else is telling you they are so sorry. I have heard and now experienced that a lot of the fight is attitude. It is easy to slip into depression. I had a good friend tell me that they were going to pull away; at least she told me in advance. Her reason was that she had lost too many people to cancer and couldn't go through losing another. I can tell you that it seriously impacted my view of what was to come for quite a while, but that was four years ago, and I am not dying any time soon.

Here is a list of things I learned the hard way, that I wish someone else had told me. First, it is okay to get a second opinion, something that honestly never even occurred to me. I had gotten to the point of wanting to give up due to chemo side effects, but I was told that the regime of chemo I was on was the only one. A good friend convinced me to go somewhere else and get a second opinion, and I found that there were other options; I no longer feel like giving in with the new regime they are using. If you are discouraged or scared, GET A SECOND OPINION.

Next, watch for the humor in the situation. Not everything in your cancer journey is going to be sad and morbid. Learn to make jokes during chemo. Gallows humor is okay. Keep an eye out for laughable moments. The more you can make fun and find things to laugh at, the better your spirits will be.

Here is another important one: it is okay to put yourself first. If you are a person that struggles with no, you need to learn it now. Over-extending during this stressful time will lead you to break down. It is okay to say I don't want to, or I can't. Blame your cancer if you need to but put yourself first. If you take care of yourself., you will be better able to be with those that you love.

If your cancer comes back after a time of remission or hiding, you DID NOT fail.

Sometimes people work hard to hide they have cancer. That gets harder when it comes back. The longer you are in rounds of chemo, the more toll it will take physically and that makes it harder to hide. Someone told me that the first round of chemo is like a battle but not the war. Until cancer has truly surrendered, you may have to fight another battle or two.

When chemo is over, you won't go back to the normal you knew before cancer. This fight changes you. Not necessarily in bad ways, but changes occur. You will need to develop a "new" normal. People get very disappointed and confused when they get off their last round of chemo and life doesn't just fall back into place.

Here is one I really wish I had been forewarned about. Chemo brain is a real thing. I will talk more about that in the chemotherapy chapter, but I will say here that it scared me for a short while. I could be in the middle of an activity and forget what I was doing. I would go to speak and struggle to recall a name or a word. Some of this is stress related and it is often reversible. I learned firsthand it is a real thing.

Do NOT sit on the internet reading up on statistical studies. You are a person not a statistic. For statistics to work, there must be some that the median does not apply to. That means on the positive end for me! Surviving cancer starts at diagnosis, not after chemo ends so stay away from the foreboding dark predictions. It affects your attitude, and as I have said - your attitude is a large part of the battle.

Your priorities will likely change, and that's okay. My priorities before cancer were focused on how to make more money. I wanted all the cool things. Now, the thing I value most is experiences. I would rather not receive more things as gifts for the most part. It turns out that my memories are the most precious thing I possess. Make memories through experiences as often as you can with the physical capabilities you have.

Fighting cancer is stressful. Having more and more things to take care of can increase this stress. Consider downsizing what you have to things that provoke/create memories and those that meet your needs. You don't have to. You don't have to do any of this. My hope is that the rest of this section will offer you ideas and suggestions. If you don't like the ones I give, perhaps it will provoke one that would work for you.

The last thing I want to leave you with is 'live for today.' No, it is not a cliché. Okay maybe it is but clichés come around because there is truth to them. No one is promised tomorrow.

You could totally be hit by a bus and not die of your diagnosis. Plan for five years from now. Know what you need to do this year to get to the five-year goals. Then live today and only today. There is a saying that if you have one foot in the past and one in the future, you will totally miss today. When your days are potentially numbered (technically every day is numbered) you need to live this one to the fullest.

Terminal Illness

If you have been given x number of months to live my heart goes out to you. The first and biggest thing I want to leave with you is not to give up hope. Remember from the previous chapter, attitude means a lot. Doctors are often right in such matters but not always. I know three people personally that were not supposed to be here today and yet they are.

One of my closest friends was told by his doctor that he would not live to see twenty-one. So, like many would do, he lived without a plan. He focused on getting as much pleasure and avoiding as much pain day to day as he could. Then one day, he woke up and realized he was thirty. As you can see, time expectations are not always correct. They are a guide, but they are not definite.

I also know two people that did indeed die from their diagnosis, however it was many years more than the doctors had predicted. One of the things I would encourage is a second opinion unless we are speaking of a few weeks.

That being said, there is no right way to process and handle a terminal diagnosis. You may be numb for a while. You may get angry. You may find yourself spiraling into depression. There is nothing wrong with a single one of these reactions. You do, however, for you own health need to take steps or get help to resolve them. You also need to forgive yourself on days that perhaps you did not handle those emotions in the way you wanted.

You may want to talk about it openly. You may want to keep it close to the chest. Whichever way you are feeling is right. If you are being quiet about it, it is still important to have someone you can talk to, even if they are the only one who knows. Being trapped in your own head can be the most dangerous place you ever walk through.

One thing to keep in mind. Those that know of your diagnosis are going to have fluctuating emotions, just like you are. They may not always react the way you want. They may have to walk away for a few minutes to gain control. This is normal for them as well. Be patient; a terminal diagnosis is hard for everyone, not just the patient.

Have your caregivers help you establish as much of a normal life routine as possible. You will have good days and bad days, which only increases the importance of living just for today. Live your day fully on the good days, and nurture and care for yourself on the bad, but having as much of your normal routine as possible will help with hope and some peace and comfort.

Doing things that are normal, routine, and often enjoyable keeps you from focusing on dying. Life should be about living these last days as fully as your health will allow. Experiences with people you love can be reassuring and maintain some peace as well.

What if you are largely alone in life? There are case managers that can help with the questions I am about to list and make arrangements for caregivers and hospice when the time comes that you need them.

There is that saying people throw about that goes 'put your affairs in order.' What the heck does that mean? On the surface, it often means a will, and people knowing whether you want to be cremated, buried, entombed etc...

Here are some other things that you might want to look at:

•	Do you have bucket list items that you can still do in the time you have? If you do, get out there and do them. I love the song that says to live like you were dying. I wish more of us did this before we know that we are indeed dying.

•	If the time comes, do you want hospice care at home or do you want to go to a facility for those passing? If you are going to leave this life, do it on your terms.

•	Are there certain things (feeding tubes, ventilator for example) that you don't want?

•	Do you have a living will or an advanced directive? These address who has the power to make decisions if you can't. It also includes if you want to be resuscitated if you start to pass.

•	Are there special belongings you want to make sure are passed to specific people? Do you want a special letter or video to go with them?

•	Is there a major project you would like to finish?

- Are there financial tasks that need to be completed? Such things might include making sure someone has your will, your life insurance policy and your bank account numbers. Do you need help with them?

This is not an inclusive list. Please add to it anything that applies to your own personal circumstance. The above items are more thought starters than anything.

As you work through this list, there may be days where you get overwhelmed or just can't deal with it emotionally. It is okay to walk away. Go nurture yourself for a bit, whether with a nap or a favorite activity. Don't feel like you must rush through a list like this. Pick the item that you feel is most important and focus on it and only it until it is done.

There is one advantage to being told you have X amount of time to live. You get to choose how your ending days are lived. You can make the arrangements in advance for how you want things to be during and after you pass. People who pass suddenly often leave many things unfinished.

The last thing I want to encourage you with is to focus on the things that enhance your life. Ask yourself, will this matter to me in a few days? Does this bring enjoyment or good memories? Does it enhance my day to day living?

What do I mean? Let me give you some examples. Many keep a journal on sites like caringbridge.com. The advantage to this is twofold. First, writing is a good way to process how you are feeling at any given moment. Secondly, friends and family can use this to stay updated on how you are doing without you having to repeat it over and over. I use this site for my own cancer fight.

In her book, <u>A Follow-Up to Watching Myself Die</u>, Karen J. Warren, Ph.D., shared her own list for enhancing your last days.

•	Save the cards, letters, emails, and text messages people send you. They are living eulogies—eulogies before you die—that you can read and enjoy now.

•	Find a support group—for you and your caregiver(s). There really is no substitute for being with others with the same challenges. And invariably, they provide helpful information of the "this is something I do" nature.

•	Write letters to your family and friends that they will have after you die. I am writing "electronic love letters" to my two grandchildren. Every few months I make a video recording for each one.

•	Plan to do something fun or pleasing each day.

- Do something new, especially if it nudges you to overcome the "What will people say?" question.

- Schedule activities to look forward to. It really makes a difference to one's mood and quality of life.

In closing, I encourage you to continue to look for the small joys. Hold your loved one's hand. Watch the sunset. Listen to the birds sing. These little joys making the days beautiful. Chris Raymond wrote, "You might not have the gift of time, but you certainly can make the most of the time that you have."

Self-Care

Yes, I know! You are already sick, so what is the point of a section on self-care? The point is that you can do nothing and be miserable, or you can do some things to make yourself feel better. One of the first things I discovered after my surgeries was that the more I didn't move, the more I didn't want to move. Then it escalated, the more I didn't move the more I couldn't move. Not bad enough, it went a step further, the more I didn't move the more depressed I became. Don't be me! (Whispers - *I got better!*)

So needless to say, the first thing I am going to tell you is MOVE! Move within the parameters that your body will allow but move. Ask your doctor what kinds of exercise would be good given your condition? What stretches are advised? Don't sit and count the days until you breathe your last. Live the most you can out of every day you have. P.S. - this philosophy works even if you are not sick!

Slow down and take time. Didn't you just tell me to move? Yes, yes I did, but I am not talking about sitting still necessarily. I am talking about time for you. Cancer or other illnesses can be overwhelming. There can be many doctor visits and treatment appointments. There can be family that is trying hard but are a bit smothering. Take some time for yourself to breathe and cope. If in that time you find yourself dropping into worry, then it is not beneficial. This should be a quiet time with a hobby: listening to music, reading a book, or processing your thoughts and feelings. In addiction counseling, I taught take one day at a time, one minute if you need to. I believe the same thing applies here. The more time you take to slow down and breathe, the calmer you will feel.

Eating: This is very important, even (maybe especially!) if you can't get much down. Hopefully your doctor has set you up with a nutritionist to address your individual needs. Your body needs food to be able to recover from treatment. Try to eat single ingredient foods as you can to avoid extra processing and preservative chemicals. Here are some general guidelines from livingbetterwith.com. It is an excellent blog for advice beyond what I have shared here.

You feel too tired to cook:

• Pre-made foods, frozen meals, or meal replacement drinks.

• Fruits and vegetables of all colors and sizes.

You feel nauseated:

• Oatmeal, crackers, plain pasta, rice and noodles.

- Ginger and peppermint. Try teas, gums, and chews.

- Cold foods, and bland foods without much scent.

- Fluids of all kinds. Keep water or high-calorie drinks on-hand. Flat Coca-Cola or ginger ale might help to minimize nausea. (Just try not to drink too close to meals – it's better to fill up on calorie-rich foods when you can than to fill your stomach with liquid).

Your sense of taste and smell has changed:

- Whatever tastes good. I mean it! What you feel like eating will change over the course of your treatment, and it's okay to listen to your body and eat whatever sounds pleasant in the moment if the portions are reasonable.

You have dry or sore mouth:

- Aim for soft foods - puddings and canned fruit and custard.

- Add sauces and gravies to your foods and avoid hot spices or sticky foods (like bread, chocolate, or peanut butter).

You're constipated:

- Head for high-fiber foods and lots and lots of liquids.

- Try adding flaxseed (linseed) to oatmeal or eating berries to boost your fiber intake.

- You should also speak to your doctor about this, as constipation caused by medication won't be improved with fiber alone.

You have diarrhea:

- Eat BRAT. BRAT stands for Bananas, Rice, Applesauce and Toast. These foods are bland and can help to settle your stomach.

You have no appetite:

- Eat in small, regular portions.

- Try protein drinks, milkshakes, smoothies, tea or soups. Sometimes, sipping on a drink is easier than eating a meal. Keep some nice liquid options and straws on-hand for the days when solid food is off the menu.

In General, Avoid These Foods During Cancer Treatment:

• High-fat or greasy fried foods. Even at the best of times, meals full of fat and grease can up-set your stomach and leave you feeling ill.

• Spicy foods. It's likely that foods with strong smells and tastes will be less appealing than plainer, blander food options. (This won't be true for everyone, so do what feels right!)

• Your favorite foods – at least right before chemo treatment. Some people recommend avoiding your favorite meals before a round of chemo, as nausea can put you off whatever you've eaten most recently.

• Magic "cure-all" cancer diets. Some people claim to have found wonderful diets that "kill cancer cells" and "shrink tumors." There is **no** scientific evidence to support these claims.

For now, you're better off eating a healthy and balanced diet, and following advice from your doctors and nurses.

As always, listen to your doctor and your body. Only you know what feels best for you!

Drink water! Water, water and more water! Those with illnesses that have nausea and fatigue are prone to dehydration. The easiest way to test if you are dehydrated is to pinch your skin. If it stays up in a tent for a second or more, you are dehydrated. Other ways to tell include dry mouth, dark urine and wrinkling of skin. Yes ladies, the first step to beauty is water!

If you feel too ill to drink liquids, suck on ice chips. The cold helps numb and yet delivers water content slowly. If you don't like water, drink what you love! Well except coffee and alcohol, these two drinks mildly contribute to dehydration. My go to when I can is watermelon. Rich in water and it doesn't feel like I am turning into a huge waterskin.

Dehydrating is easy enough due to nausea. If you have other symptoms such as vomiting or diarrhea, it becomes a bigger problem. Make sure you talk to your doctor about these symptoms and increase liquid intake. Dehydration has continued to be one of the big factors and problems in my cancer fight. The base recommendation is 68 ounces a day, *before* you add other side effects and weight differences. If you are not getting at least 8 eight-ounce glasses of liquid (other than coffee and alcohol), you need to work on this. Water is also beneficial to brain functioning and helps fight fatigue. The body begins to slow down when it is low on water. Those need for frequent naps or cups of coffee could just be your body crying out for water. Studies have shown that even a 1% decrease in water levels can affect mood and energy.

These three things, (moving, water and nutrition) are necessary for you to feel the best you can in your fight. Remember, the focus is to get the most out of our days. Eat what you need, not what others like. Take those moments to yourself to recharge and move even if it is leg lifts in bed.

I want to speak to one other physical manifestation or side effect of some medications, neuropathy. My first experience with this began with a medicine called Oxaliplatin. The doctor had warned me about an extreme painful reaction to cold and he was not kidding. I couldn't even touch things coming out of the freezer. When I was done with this medication, I couldn't feel very well with my fingers and toes and I had pins and needles every time I touched something. There are medications to help with this and I am still on them today.

If you don't feel it is bad enough to be on a long-term medication, there are some over the counter treatments that will help milder neuropathy.

• Non-steroidal anti-inflammatory drugs (NSAIDs), such as ibuprofen, may help control pain. These are available over the counter.

• Topical ointments and creams, such as capsaicin 0.075 percent cream, containing chili pepper, may ease pain. Patches are also available.

Ask your doctor to check your vitamin D levels, especially if you are also depressed. Low vitamin D has been shown to increase both depression and neuropathy.

Low levels of Vitamin B6 and B12 can also contribute to this pain. However, most people get what they need from these two vitamins through food. Cancer patients have a history of not eating properly so this is something to keep in mind.

A hot bath is my favorite one. I feel like neuropathy is on every nerve ending some days. A hot bath does wonders to lower my stress and ease this discomfort on bad days. If mobility is an issue, make sure you have someone who can help you get out. One time I almost didn't make it out of the tub successfully. BE CAREFUL!

Advocate for yourself and ask questions, be a part of treatment decisions. I am going to share one other thing, if you have a caregiver, take them into appointments with you. Your caregivers can spot things you may have forgotten or haven't noticed in the face of other things. It is okay to let them in on your full situation, it really is.

But back to one of my first points - get moving! Increased blood flow helps with this pain and healing. Oh, and guess what - cigarettes reduce blood flow to these small nerves, so you might want to consider stopping that if it is a habit.

All this being said, always speak to your doctor and if his advice is different than my sharing of personal information and experience - LISTEN TO YOUR DOCTOR FIRST!

Social Care

Social Care? Why are you talking about social care? My answer: it is necessary. For many people the first instinct is to curl up inside yourself; I know this firsthand. There is this mindset that is easy to fall into. "If I push them all away, it will be easier for them when I pass." It isn't true. Logically it should be, but it is not.

Instead of pulling in, push out. If you are an introvert, then only do it for a short while at a time. There is nothing wrong at a family gathering with pulling away for a while to catch your breath or recenter. If you are an extrovert, then this will probably be easy for you if you let go of the 'push them away' mentality.

"I don't know what to say? Everyone wants to talk about my diagnosis." Diseases like cancer tend to take over our lives. It is difficult to focus outside of it. The easiest answer to this is to ask questions and just listen. How is your family? What is new in your life? These kinds of questions, followed by just listening and asking additional questions to keep the conversation moving helps the other person to also move past your diagnosis.

Another thing you need to have in your life is something you are passionate about that is also not controversial. This allows you to share excitement and again, talk about something other than your diagnosis. Are you into animals, current events, or volunteering? It doesn't matter what it is, just pick something that interests you and learn all you can about it. Eventually someone is going to ask questions back, and you need to have something to talk about. Try to avoid politics and religion. These never seem to end well at gatherings or if you and the other person share opposing views.

Develop a support system. You can join a support group in your community for similar diagnoses or create one through family and friends. A lot of people are going to ask you what you need. Your number one answer should be someone to talk to now and then. Pick those you know will really listen and be there for you. This group of friends and family will become your lifeline to sanity.

The benefit to a community support group is that it normalizes your diagnosis. There is a condition called "terminal uniqueness." Basically, it means you think you are the only one and so you remain quiet and it is killing you. In a community support group, you know that other people understand what you are feeling and help suggest and share ways to overcome the problems your diagnosis.

Believe it or not, this one area of focus, socializing, can help reduce tumors. According to a research study reported on by Matthew Moore, "Cancer patients who change their lifestyle to keep company with more people could see substantial improvements in their condition, the study suggests."

Limiting our social interactions also contributes to depression. Isolation leaves you in your own head, and in many cases, this is the most dangerous place a person can be. It is easy to fall into feeling sorry for one's self. The simplest social interactions can divert our attention outside ourselves.

Is laughter really the best medicine? There are many studies to support that it is. Laughter brightens your day and lifts your spirits contributing to a better overall mindset. I really suggest you make socializing a priority once you are over the first heavy shock of hearing you have a lifelong disease. You owe it to yourself and your health to be with others so you can share joys, struggles and laughter. Even better, it really does strengthen you for the fight to come.

Intellectual Care

Let's talk about chemo brain, also known as chemo fog. First, there is no scientific proof that chemo alone causes this. Despite researchers inability to confirm its name, all agree that chemo brain is something many cancer fighters experience. The Mayo Clinic posted this list of symptoms.

Signs and symptoms of chemo brain may include the following:

- Being unusually disorganized
- Confusion
- Difficulty concentrating
- Difficulty finding the right word
- Difficulty learning new skills
- Difficulty multitasking

- Fatigue
- Feeling of mental fogginess
- Short attention span
- Short-term memory problems
- Taking longer than usual to complete routine tasks
- Trouble with verbal memory, such as remembering a conversation
- Trouble with visual memory, such as recalling an image or list of words

I am not sure if this is true of other life-threatening illnesses, but I can confirm from personal experience that for cancer, this is a real phenomenon. It can cause a sense of lost intelligence and confusion. Things that were easy sometimes get harder without any explanation.

So, what do you do about it? Well first, stop trying to multitask. Most cases of chemo brain are just not up for it. Instead, practice mindfulness. What is mindfulness? There are whole books about this, but I will give you a simplified version.

It is focusing everything about you into the moment. It does not include letting the past or future intrude on that moment. Whatever you are doing, put your full mind and senses into it. Listening to children? listen with your full attention. Doing the dishes? feel the sensation of the water and really focus on doing the dishes well. Our society has pushed this idea that multitasking is the way to go. Studies have shown that it increases productivity if you can focus fully on the task at hand. Yoga is a good way to learn to do this. You are focused on a specific pose, how your body feels in that moment and paying attention to its physical messages. By the way, this lowers stress levels as well.

The next thing you can do is what health professionals emphasize constantly: Eat right, move, and get sleep. You may need help with the sleep part if your mind can't let go of your worries. There is no shame in this.

Challenge your brain is my next tip. Do puzzles, word games, chess. Anything that makes you slow down, but also makes you think. Some people like TED talks for this stimulation, other people love doing jigsaw puzzles for their brain challenge. Just make sure it is something you enjoy.

Establish routines. This way when your brain just refuses to come to your call, some things are on autopilot. Take your medicines at the same time or moment each day. For example, I take three sets of meds four times a day. I have timed them with breakfast, lunch, dinner and bed. This helps me remember to take them. The more you can put your life into a routine the easier it will be to remember things. Don't overdo this though, you want it to be a routine not a rut.

Use tools. There is nothing wrong with Post-It notes, calendars, and reminder apps. This works well for commitments that are out of your routines. A doctor's visit, a social call, or anything else unusual.

The last one is asking for help. Despite cultural norms about asking for help, it does not make you weak. You have an illness. I have already encouraged you to create a support system. If you are struggling with anything that is becoming a pattern or continued problem, ask for help. Don't wait till something bad comes of it. Ask for help the moment you realize there is a problem regardless of what category it comes from. Mental health care is important in any major disease; heck for anyone to be honest. The first thing I encourage you to do is go outside! In most cases, this will help you feel a bit better within minutes. There is vitamin D from the sun.

Fresh air circulating through your system and something outside your four walls.

Take a sense walk. Find somewhere away from the house, even if it is down the street a few houses to a bench. Stand or sit, close your eyes, and listen. What do you hear? Feel - What do you feel? Sun or wind on your face, your feet in your shoes. Hear - What do you hear? Go deeper, what is beyond the first sounds. Open your eyes - What do you see?

Do this exercise with mindfulness. It can lower stress, calm anger and reduce anxiety for many. It costs you nothing and is easy to do any-where. Please don't close your eyes standing if you have a history of falling over, though!

Tell people that you don't need any more things. Make this a point. If you are facing end of life, you are probably trying to give some of these things away. Tell them you are more interested in experiences. Make memories instead of obtaining treasures. Share your bucket list with your support system. Start with the easiest one first just to get moving on these. Even simpler, try different restaurants with friends and family. Explore different parks or just sit and laugh over tea/coffee.

The final thing I want to talk about is grieving. If you have been told you have a life-threatening or changing illness, you are going to need to grieve. Some of the things you might need to grieve is loss of mobility, independence or life goals you had set. It is okay to go through the grieving process, but once you reach acceptance, let it go.

Now is the time to get the best out of every day you can. To sum up: Eat, move, sleep, challenge your brain, make memories and get out there.

Spiritual Care

"Why are you talking about religion?" "I am angry at God and this topic makes me angry too." Woah... Woah… Woah. I am not talking about a higher power or religion. Let's get that straight right out the door. Can spiritual care include your personal faith and higher power? Of course, but it does not have to.

It is a fact that many people have a faith, but they are also angry at their higher power. They shake their fists and ask, "Why me?" or "How could you let this happen?" A life-threatening illness can bring up a lot of feelings of anger and betrayal at the beginning. So, for the rest of this thread, we are going to leave your relationship with your higher power to you. There is no way I can speak to this without stepping on someone's toes.

"Well then what do you mean?" I mean taking care of that inner "I". People call it by many names. I have heard soul, spirit, firing neurons and life force. Whatever you believe it is, one thing is universal: scientists cannot dissect a corpse and find it. That uniqueness that makes you... well, you… needs taken care of and nourished.

In the study, <u>Spiritual Needs of Cancer Patients: A Qualitative Study</u>, researchers concluded that spiritual needs of cancer patients should be recognized, realized, and considered in care of patients by the medical team. An all-out support of health system policy makers to meet patients' spiritual needs is particularly important. That is a pretty bold statement.

According to Florence Nightingale's philosophy of care, spirituality is inherent in humans and is the deepest and strongest source of healing. Thus, one of the nurses' responsibilities is attention to spiritual dimensions of care and providing a healing ambience for patients. See, I am not making this stuff up. So, how? Let's delve into that, as holistic care has shown stronger results than symptomatic care. Four themes came out of the study: connection, seeking peace, meaning/purpose and transcendence. So, let's look at the first one, connection.

Connection. What is the importance of connection? I have already touched on this by sharing that one should get out and not isolate, but let's dig a little deeper. Connection doesn't just mean with other people. It is also talking about with one's self. If you cannot connect and love yourself, you will become needy by seeking it in others so desperately that they push away. This confirms that inner thought that "I am not lovable." If you can connect with that "I" within you and love who it is, the ability to provide love to yourself and others creates a great sense of fulfillment. I recommend a book called <u>Inner Bonding: Self-Healing Process</u> by Margaret Paul, Ph.D.; you can pick it up at http://www.innerbonding.com/

There is a Vivian Green quote I love around seeking peace. "Life isn't about waiting for the storm to pass, it's about learning to dance in the rain." There are several things you can do to seek that inner peace. The first thing is to learn to trust yourself. Your intuition is a self-guide harvested by the "I" from experience and just gut instinct. Take one day at a time and just focus on making that day the best it can be. Don't compare it to other days. Some days are better than others. Just make today the best it can be.

Another thing you can do is ease your expectations. Let's face it, there is no guarantee of an easy ride in this life. You are also ill. You can't expect the same things of yourself that you would prior to being ill. Slow down a little, focus on each moment, and breathe. You must see and accept things as they are instead of as you hoped or expected them to be. Create a new normal for yourself that is a little less demanding.

Next, have hope. A road centered on hope is far more enjoyable than a road of despair. Could it end badly? It could. But living every moment you have with an attitude of hope makes whatever journey is before you pleasant to travel. Gain a sense of balance and hope for the best, it will make living each day to the fullest much easier and pleasurable.

Move towards what you want rather than running away from what you don't want. Angel Chernoff wrote that "By persistently trying to move away from what you don't want, you are forced to think about it so much that you end up carrying its weight along with you. But if you instead choose to focus your energy on moving toward something you do want, you naturally leave the negative weight behind as you progress forward." These are just a few suggestions for working peace of mind. There are many books out there that focus on just this area of your spirituality -- seeking peace.

Finding purpose. I am going to give you a step by step process for finding your purpose. But answer these questions in the here and now. Not before cancer. Right now.

1. What are your strengths right now? What do others say you do well?

2. Don't settle. Just because you have a life-threatening illness does not mean you now have to just take what is given to you.

3. Try - action is not optional. You must get out there and try different things to find out what you can do with any new limitations you find yourself now experiencing. You must try things that can work around those limitations as well.

4.   It is finding purpose in this new life situation that helps you continue to live with passion. Your purpose will not be work. It will drive you to get up in the morning and move when you are feeling like curling up into a ball.

Are you doing what you love, what energizes you, and gives you deep fulfillment? If not, what are you waiting for?

Transcendence is rising above our material-oriented world. It is that moment when life is not about that next new toy. You look around your home and realize that you have way too many things. Things take up energy and clutter our homes. Then we must dust and keep these many things serviceable and put up. It is a lot of spent energy. Energy better used in your purpose and maintaining your support system/friends and family.

Some other things that you can do to help that spiritual side includes setting a morning and evening ritual. There is comfort in rituals to help you get moving and to relax and wind down at the end of the day.

Part of that evening ritual should be to sit with yourself for just few minutes and just mentally list every piece of the day that you loved. Example: I loved sitting by the window and just watching it rain, I loved my granddaughter's laugh when we played, etc. Take a moment. How can you build more of what you loved into your routines or daily experiences?

Occasionally, write yourself a letter and make sure to list out what you love doing and what you don't like doing. List out what you should be saying no to or saying yes to. What have I learned about myself, work, or the world? Writing these letters, a couple times a month not only leaves a record of your path through your illness, it is a guide to improve future days as well. Occasionally you should sit down and read the last few. It will help you focus on living life rather than living in despair.

The last thing I want to refocus you on is engaging your senses. Make sure you give your eyes beautiful things to look at. When you go to quiet places, take a moment and run through the appropriate senses. What do you hear, see, feel, or smell? Are you eating? focus in on the taste and really savor it. Make this an activity on days that you are fixated on a negative thought. It often helps one to break free of repetitive negative thinking.

This list of ideas is nowhere close to exhaustive, but I hope they will at least inspire other ideas that you can to nourish your inner self. You need to respond to your own needs and feel balanced as you can in the face of the stress of illness.

Lastly, a brief touch on religious values. There is a difference between believing in a higher power and following the dictates of a specific religion. Every religion will say it is the right one. If you are looking for a higher power connection, stay with the one you feel the that inner spirit responds to in a nourishing and encouraged way.

Why do I bring this up? According to the US Centers for Disease Control and Prevention (CDC), 69% of cancer patients say they pray for their health. A recent study published in Cancer, a peer-reviewed journal of the American Cancer Society, suggests a link between religious or spiritual beliefs and better physical health reported among patients with cancer.

Whatever path you take, it is a known fact that meditating, getting out in nature, spending time with loved ones, and volunteering are all associated with positive health benefits. This is largely to do with spiritual self-care and personal meaning to life. Don't ignore this area of your wellbeing. Strong positive attitudes are known to help fight against illness and are known to come from balance of the mind, emotions,physical and spiritual self-care.

Letter to Caregivers

Dear Caregivers,

Thank you! Thank you for all you do and are trying to do. Without you, those of us in advance stages of our disease could not have any life satisfaction. I know those that have been a caregiver for me over the last four years will have my enduring love and gratitude.

Many patients today receive a lot of their care at home. Things that used to be done in hospitals are now completed at home, largely because it has been found that people recover better in their own environment. This care is provided by spouses, partners, children, other relatives, and family friends.

There are some things that I have observed watching caregivers, and some of these may not apply to you. But generally, it is good advice to have in your pocket. The first is, don't enable us to languish. It is easy to slip into depression, curl up on the couch and not move, but moving is important. Doing the things we can do for ourselves is important. (UNLESS DOCTOR HAS SAID OTHERWISE) Don't let your friend or family member stop doing things for themselves if you know they are capable. It seems like it is nurturing and loving, but it is damaging. Not to say that you can't do that now and then out of love and respect, just don't let it be how the two of you interact on a common basis.

Moving reduces symptoms and improves physical capacity, which in turn is expected to improve daily functioning. There is research supporting this in several places. If the not moving continues, it really does impact our ability to do things; at one point I was losing my ability to walk. Sometimes occupational therapy can help; I learned to move and walk again naturally despite my disease. This in turn lifted my mood and began a life turnaround.

The next thing I would like to share with you is that you need to advocate for your friend/family member. That said, it is important to remember that there is a difference between advocating and making decisions for your patient who is ill. Make sure that you both understand the diagnosis, have talked about the risks and benefits of treatment options, and then let the patient choose their path. It can be hard to do this if you don't agree with the choice, but ultimately, it needs to be the patient's decision until a power of attorney is enacted. Even then, you should try to adhere to what you know the friend/family member wished to happen.

Ask questions! There was a time when a patient was diagnosed, told what the treatment will be and then the patient would just follow through. That has changed. Patients are encouraged to work with their doctor and know what to report. Keep a notepad around so that you or your friend/family member can write down important but not urgent questions for each visit.

Sometimes the doctor will ask questions and as the patient, we say we don't think so. With chemo brain, it is totally possible to have or not have a symptom the doctor is asking about, and helpful when the caregiver can gently correct the answer. Make sure you and the patient have discussed you going into

appointments beforehand and why it would be helpful.

If things seem off to you or there are complications, help your patient get a second opinion. Let me share my example: I was losing my ability to walk. My oncologists kept me supplied with pain killers to deal with the pain of moving. When I got to the Mayo clinic for my second opinion, however, it turned out that my increasing inability to move and stand had nothing to do with my cancer. Instead, I had bursitis that had been allowed to progress to severe levels. I would have never almost lost my ability to walk if I had gotten the second opinion sooner. If anything seems off or too dramatized, get a second opinion. If it is life threatening, encourage the patient to take the treatment offered until you can get a second opinion. It can take some time to set up a second opinion appointment.

Verbal Support: I want to give you some things not to do when attempting to give moral support. Don't compare your friend/family member's journey to another. It is not helpful to hear - "Oh my grandma had that, she died." Nope... not helpful at all.

Don't ask 'How are you?' unless you really want to know and are ready to respect the patient's avoidance if they don't want to answer it. Nine times out of ten you are going to get - "I am fine," when they are not. Don't say, "You got this!" You don't know that. Cancer can be virulent and when facing that statement, the first thought as a patient is "you don't know that" or "no I don't." It also discounts the ill person's own very real fears or sad feelings.

So, what do you say to someone with a life altering disease? Respond from your heart! Instead of saying "how can I help?" which can be an overwhelming question, offer what you can do. "If you need help with _______ call me" is a good way to phrase this. If you are good at listening, offer yourself to the ill person with something along the lines of "Hey, if you just need to talk, call me." Sometimes just offering to take the dog out now and then is such a stress relief to the patient.

One of the most common questions I get is 'what do I say when I first learn someone has cancer?' A good one is, "I am sorry you have to go through that." Try to avoid just "I am so sorry," it brings up the question of "for what?" Another good one is "I'm not sure what to say, but I want you to know I care," or "I'll keep you in my thoughts/prayers."

Allow the ill person to find humor in their disease. Laughter is good and dark humor can be a good way of processing out those feelings that are so overwhelming. If you find the humor hard to listen to, then you need someone to talk to as well. Which leads me to the next major area of support.

Self-care. I know I did a section for the patient on self-care. I am not talking to the patient right now. I am talking to you! You cannot help your friend/family member if you don't have anything left to give. Think of it like this, in a power outage your phone will still have power for some time. Eventually if power is not restored that battery runs out and there is nothing left to give. The same thing happens to caregivers. They care and care, give and give, then find themselves snapping at people, exhausted or just wanting to quit.

Being a caregiver can be exhausting both physically and emotionally. With every new symptom there is that little bird in the back of your mind that goes, "Is this it?" Watching someone you love struggle is draining before you even start doing things to help them. Then there are the many appointments, recovery from surgeries, medications, meals, schedules, and health insurance matters. It can be overwhelming.

Here are some common tips: Eat well-balanced meals and do so on a regular schedule.

Take a daily multivitamin. Drink six to eight glasses of water a day.

Move every day: Move your body daily, even if it's simply 15 minutes of stretching, yoga, calisthenics or walking. Use the stairs to keep your circulation going.

Get outdoors: Fresh air renews the body and spirit — even if you only have time for a brief outing. When possible, open a window.

Get your sleep: Strive for a minimum of seven to eight hours of consecutive sleep in a those 24-hour period. Nap when your loved one naps.

Watch your own health: That is, get treatments for your own aches and pains before they turn into something more serious.

Don't ignore your emotions: Pay attention to your own feelings and emotions, and seek counseling or caregiver support groups if needed.

Vent feelings to trusted family members or friends.

Take a break: Have a friend or family member sit with your family member if they can't be alone for a time. Use relaxation or stress management methods such as meditation, visualization and yoga. Books and videos are available to guide you in these techniques.

Get positive input: There are helpful magazines like Today's Caregiver or Caring Today. My favorite is Chicken Soup for the Caregiver's soul. If you are religious, keep in touch with your faith-based activities.

Chuckle more often: It is true, laughter is good medicine. Laugh, reminisce and share stories of happy times.

Ask for help: Friends, family and religious groups may be eager to assist and are only waiting to be asked and directed. Doing everything yourself deprives others of an opportunity to feel like they have helped where they could. Don't be a martyr.

If the patient in your life needs care most of the day check into your state. Some states will allow a family member to be paid to provide care. These benefits and rates of pay vary wildly from state to state. If not for you, sometimes they will pay the person who is giving you a break for coming in while you work or just take a break. It is at least worth investigating.

Please, please take care of yourself. You can't help the ill person if you are not well. And know this, you are loved and appreciated even if the person is lashing out now and then. We could not make this difficult journey without you. You are, well, our life preserver.

Thank you!

Cheri Matthynssens

Letter to Family and Friends

Dear Family and Friends,

You are allowed to have feelings about cancer. Cancer doesn't just affect the patient, it impacts everyone around them. We hear the word cancer and we immediately think they are dying. Panic ensues and all the other emotions that go with it. Breathe!

This letter is to those that are not the actual caregivers. Often, I am told, "I don't know how to help," so here are some ideas. First, if you are close enough, offer to give the caregiver a break. Pick up groceries for them or sit with your loved one while the caregiver gets out for a bit. Caregivers are often under the assumption that they must do it all alone stoically. They might not ask for help, offer it anyway.

One caregiver I spoke to mentioned that she wished someone would have just offered a bed for a night away before her loved one needed her 24/7. You would be surprised how this one thing alone will help a lot. There are so many things you can do even if you can't be the actual caregiver. Offer to come over and help deep clean the house, mow the yard, or other things that might get neglected due to appointments, health management and side effects. Sometimes, just your presence is support enough.

However you can help, be specific. A lot of times, people will say "let me know if you need anything," but when the patient or caregiver needs something, they are afraid to ask. What if their need is not what you were thinking of when you offered? Also, some people say those words but are counting on not being asked. So instead you can offer things like: "If you need to talk, I can make a cup of coffee. If you need help getting to appointments, I can help." This kind of specific offer sets a clear expectation about what things you feel most qualified to help with.

Offer more than once. Caregivers are notorious for not asking for help and feeling all alone. Eventually, they will reach out if they know the offer was sincere. If they just want to talk, they may not need advice. Just listen, ask questions to show you are listening and reassure them they are not alone. If they ask for advice, *then* offer it.

Too far away to help in that way? Can you help financially with things like paying a landscape company to keep the lawn mowed, or a housekeeping service? Little things add up; even sending a new jigsaw puzzle or craft supplies if you know the patient enjoys that activity can make a big difference. For example, I spend a great deal of time painting acrylics. Really it can even go a step simpler. Send an amusing or supportive card once in a while. Call up and really listen. Your support here and there means a lot to the caregiver and the patient.

You can expect changes from the person with the illness. Medications, fear, and side effects can often lead to depression or lashing out. Hold your boundaries firmly but gently, but also understand that the stress of all that they are going through is the root of this behavior change. Another change often experienced is loss of memory. In cancer, we call this chemo brain. Bottom line, there will be good and bad days.

It is very important not to offer false optimism. Things like you will beat this or you got this have a huge risk of not being true. When someone says you got this to me, I immediately think, "No I don't." Be real and honest. Say things like, I am sorry you have to go through this.

If your family member wants to talk about their death or arrangements, don't put them off by saying something like that isn't going to happen. Many patients report a feeling of relief when these things are taken care of and no longer a stressor. Some patients deal with their emotions around cancer with gallows humor. Just know it is their way of processing how they are feeling, and there is nothing wrong with it. Take your cues from the ill person. Some people are very private and don't want to talk about it, others need to talk; some can joke, and some cannot. Follow their lead.

The most important thing I can leave you with is to try and keep things as normal as possible. While some gentling may be in order, keep your boundaries and routines. If you went out to tea on Saturdays, still offer tea on Saturdays. Maybe it needs to be at their house now, but when you can keep routines as normal as possi-

ble, it is reassuring to the person that is ill.

A Letter to Professionals

Dear Professionals, i.e. nurses, doctors and palliative care.

Thank you! I cannot thank you enough for giving me more days to my life and life to my days. That being said, there are some things I would like to share with you.

As many of you probably guessed, you are the lifeline between our home lives and our medical lives. Some of us don't have strong support systems; you are it. You are the only one to listen to our fears, problems, hopes and dreams. I know it must get overwhelming at times, so many of us sharing these things amidst your many other duties, but we need you to. I think the day I felt most supported was when my physician's assistant really listened and took steps to fix a problem on the medical team's side. I didn't feel as alone.

The issue that the PA helped with was being treated like a number, so that is the next thing I wish to share. I know oncology and other departments are helping dozens of people daily, but we are still people. We are still scared of dying, in pain, and terrified of the treatments that bring side effects and sometimes more pain. Try to remember that this is a human sitting there and not a training dummy.

Watch where you talk about your medical patients. Not just for HIPPA reasons, but because what is overheard can be misunderstood. I don't want to know about Ms. Smith's medical issues or how close to death Mr. Jones is. Sometimes we can hear things about ourselves. Once I was in the hospital and I heard a nurse tell another that I needed moved to another room because I was a dirty patient. Today, I know what that means. But partially sedated, I heard that I needed a bath and was someone to avoid. It took ten minutes for my caregiver to help me settle my overstrung emotional response.

Please don't say you understand what we are going through. Unless you have sat in that chair with the same diagnosis, you don't know. You may empathize, but there is no way you can know. There is more to us than our diagnosis, so every little bit of that interacts with what we are going through.

Don't discount our concerns. There is nothing worse than be told over and over that "I am sure it is nothing," only to find out is everything. I will continue to use my own experience as examples. I saw four doctors over five months and kept getting told it was nothing. I knew deep down that something was horribly wrong with how my digestive system was working and how I was feeling. By the time a doctor really listened to me, the consulting surgeon said I was weeks from death. It should not be like that. Yes, I know some people are hypochondriacs. Don't treat all of us like one.

Don't hide behind your years of training to discount our fears or concerns. There is nothing worse than being talked down to while you are sitting there terrified. More than once I experienced the situation where I felt like the doctor was saying "I know everything." and that I was being stupid for advocating for myself. We are taught to advocate for ourselves in almost every major illness support group.

Please don't say "you will be fine." You don't have a crystal ball. I have heard nurses say that. My first question is 'how can you be sure?' Things can go wrong with the simplest of procedures. Once I had a full body reaction to the cleansing clothes that they use before surgery. Weird things happen. It also comes across as placating at a time when most patients are seeking truth. I know you think it sounds reassuring, but when one is dealing with a severe illness, it just creates doubt in your truthfulness.

Please use layman's terms. I know you are smart, it is why I came to see you. But when explaining my care, I need to understand it. Also, why you are recommending a certain path over other paths of care. What makes this recommendation the best for me? These are things we need to know.

Please don't be insulted if I ask for a second opinion. Two sets of eyes on a situation are always better than one. Also, a lot of times this is us, as patients, not wanting to hear what you are telling us. Let us get that out of our system and if that was the problem, we will be back. It is reassuring when two professionals come up with the same conclusion and recommendations.

Understand that severe illness comes with price tags: some emotional, some physical, and most always financial. My chemo costs $17K a dose. I have heard people shrug and say your insurance covers it. They don't know the sheer terror that drives you to sacrifice anything and everything to make sure you can pay your insurance, deductibles, and copays. For those of us on disability, we are often paying two insurance premiums. Cancer has taken everything from me on a financial level. When people must have Go-FundMe accounts just to stay alive. Needless to say, they are in a bit of distress. Then along comes someone sharing one more thing that has a price tag.

My ex-husband had a heart attack with no insurance. The hospital wouldn't work with him on payments at a level he could afford so they sold his account to a debt collector. That debt collector got a court order to take so much monthly that he lost the home the kids had known all their life. So, please know that the moment our lives touch yours, unless we are affluent, our lives just got harder.

Lastly, please don't tell us to calm down. This often come after being told something that is about to totally upend our life. Disbelief and panic set in almost immediately. If you were told that your license was suspended, you would be a little upset. Sorry, that is the closest comparison I could make without knowing you.

All this being said, thank you for the years in school, the time in my life and the care and concern that almost every one of you shows. For many of us, we would not still be upright on this world without you.

My Story

I think about my story and I have to wonder about divine providence. So many times, doors opened that I would have never thought possible. It all started in February of 2014. I had been having some intestinal issues that were just not abating. I remember soaking in the tub one night as this seemed to ease the discomfort and thinking, "I have cancer." The thought prompted a call to the clinic that I was attached to and an appointment.

The doctor assured me it was probably nothing but did some routine tests for intestinal challenges. She called back and reassured me that as she suspected, it was nothing. So another month passed, and I went back still feeling no better. I was told again, it was probably nothing but a couple more tests were done to rule out some typical intestinal issues. Again, I got the call, "It is nothing."

I poured myself into my fantasy fiction writing and began to make a name for myself. I was selling an average of 350 eBooks a day. Given my health, I began to wonder if my illness was stress related. As my writing was successful enough to pay the bills, I gave notice at my job.

During this same period of time I was not improving. I started eating foods like soup and applesauce, things that were gentle to my system. Nothing seemed to help. Finally, the symptoms became alarming and I made another appointment. My regular doctor was busy, so I got in to see a PA. It was a man I knew, who had at one time worked at the clinic that I was attached to as an addiction counselor. My first words were something is horribly wrong, and no one is listening. He did his exam and left the room. When he returned, he informed me that he had run my symptoms past the surgeon in the building, and they wanted me to make an immediate appointment to see this surgeon.

I met with the surgeon, and he was deeply concerned. He scheduled a colonoscopy for just a couple days later. I went into that appointment relieved that someone was listening, but I was not expecting the outcome. Beside the fact that I had told myself in February that I had cancer, hearing those words from the surgeon as I came to in recovery created emotions I cannot describe. The surgeon told me that the cancer was so advanced that he had been unable to scope past it, and that I had been within weeks - if not days - of a complete blockage. He scheduled the surgery to remove it as soon as possible.

This was a complete upheaval of my life. Only those that have been diagnosed with a potentially terminal illness can truly understand all the fears, emotions and pure panic that sweeps through you simultaneously. I had no idea which way to turn or what to do.

The surgery did not go as planned. They took one-third of my colon and found the cancer in four lymph nodes. Then, the actual wound and resection did not heal correctly. They went in three times through the same incision. One of those times was to clean out the cut as it picked up MRSA in the hospital. Finally, all the surgeries were done, and I was sent to an oncologist.

Due to it only being in four lymph nodes they were fairly certain they had caught it in time before it spread. I did six months of chemother-apy and was in a pretty good space. I wrote my most popular novel from the chemo chair. I had a positive outlook and was not overly concerned. Unfortunately, during this time there were indica-tions that a kidney wasn't functioning properly.

So, when chemotherapy was complete, I went to have that looked at.

It turned out that in one of the three colon surgeries, my ureter had been nicked and scarred. I did six months of chemotherapy with a blocked kidney. It was very damaged. First, they tried to reboot it, as it was only functioning at 8%. I had a tube in my back for three months to try to kick start the kidney. They tried to put a stent in it, but it was too damaged. Finally, we made the decision to remove it so it didn't later cause problems.

I had been home three days from the kidney surgery with stitches around about a third of my body when a wildfire changed directions and headed straight for our hobby farm. We had been somewhat prepacked just in case, but I was home alone when this happened. I called for help and was working to load up last minute things. During this, I felt a horrible tearing and was scared I had popped internal stitches. So once our things and animals were safe, I went to the E.R. While the kidney wound was undamaged, they found a 9 cm tumor on my ovary. Here I was, trying to deal with the fear of my home burning down, when I learned the cancer had metastasized. It was back.

Once I had recovered enough from the kidney surgery, they scheduled a surgery to remove the ovary. If it turned out to be a genetic match to the original cancer, they would do a full hysterectomy. It matched. By this time, I was sick of surgeries.

I started a second round of chemo and was on it for about six months. It was unpleasant. The therapy induced such a sensitivity to cold, I couldn't touch things from the freezer with my bare hands. Winters in Okanogan County are very cold, so going outside was a miserable experience. The worst part though, was that I couldn't eat ice cream. No one should have to give up ice cream! But I weathered it, and life began to return to normal.

It didn't last long. After about five months off chemo, the cancer came back, this time in my liver. I was an hour and a half from my oncologist at this point. The hobby farm had burned, and though the house had survived, the constant dust had become unmanageable. I convinced my caregiver and partner to move to the city my oncologist was in. There would be no dust. We would be close to the hospital and I would feel safer. There had been a couple trips the previous winter due to severe side effects that had been made in snow storms and had been frightening.

This was the worst mistake I could have made. It was good for me, but it destroyed my partner. He had left a job he felt good doing. He gave up the farm he had wanted all his life. We left our horses and goats behind. He fell into a deep depression. He needed to go back, but he wouldn't without me. He couldn't find decent work in the town we moved to, and it was pulling him down deeper into that depression. Again, I didn't know what to do. I completed chemotherapy and had a liver resection to pull out the last obstinate tumor.

The hardest part for me, besides watching my partner's decline, was that I couldn't talk about it to anyone else. My kids didn't want to talk about my cancer. They didn't want to talk about the potential terminal threat over my head. It was then that my social worker suggested I write this book. I let it drop and percolate but did not return to the idea for over a year.

This next migration of my cancer did not take much of a break. Within a couple of months, it was in my lungs. I had reached the point where quantity of life was beginning to outweigh quality, and I was considering giving up.

A good friend and his wife convinced me to move Minnesota and get treatment at the Mayo Clinic. It was a horrible decision for me to have to make. I knew my partner was not going to get better by going with me, so I made the decision to push him away. I knew it hurt him horribly, but now looking back, it was the right decision. He returned to his previous employer and is focused and productive.

Again, I downsized. We had gone from a three-bedroom farm home to a 980 ft apartment in the first move. This time, I was going to drive to Minnesota with only what my car could carry. Reducing your life's memories and belongings to a carload is not a situation I wish on anyone. Due to my poor health, my daughter went with me to make sure I could make the drive all the way there.

By this time, I could barely walk. The oncologist had said the joint pain was due to side effects of chemo and kept me supplied in pain medication. My friends received me into their home in the worst shape I had been in since the cancer journey started.

I set up my consultation with the Mayo Clinic, and it was encouraging. They had different options from the chemo I had been on, which would allow my quality of life to return. They discovered that my inability to walk had nothing to do with side effects. I had a case of bursitis that had been allowed to progress to severe levels. I was soon set up with chemo, as well as physical therapy with palliative and physical care doctors on my team.

In three months, I was walking again. It was about this time that my outlook at life began to swing. I had spent the last three and half years fighting cancer. It had never once occurred to me to learn to live with the fight. Slowly, other things began to return to my focus. I learned to have a life despite cancer. My positive focus began to return and with it, a me that I was proud of sharing with others.

I am not going to share that everything is perfect. It isn't. My cancer has begun growing while ON chemo. I am not giving up, but the fight is escalating. However, my inner peace has never been stronger. My hopes and dreams are stronger than they have ever been. I am planning a life for five years down the road. Cancer may be within me, but it no longer defines me. I hope this journey leads you to the same place. Life lived in bitterness is no way to live.

Conclusion

I hope you have found this small book helpful. It was very cleansing to write it and I know that if I had been given such a book when my journey started, I would have had an easier time of it.

My hope for you is that you can avoid some of the pitfalls that my caregiver and I experienced. Living in depression and thinking of dying all the time is no way to live. No one knows how many days they have on this planet. Even having been given a year to live does not mean that one is now exempt from car accidents, other ailments or just plain bad luck.

Even if you are not sick as you read this, live its principles and you will be happier and healthier in life. My best wishes to every one of you.

Namastes

About the Author

Cheryl Matthynssens was born in Upland, California, has held a teaching degree and was a licensed addictions counselor and sales manager. This has allowed her to interview hundreds of personalities over her career.

She loves that everyone is unique, and this appreciation and interest has informed and inspired her writing.

Matthynssens enjoys the universe of fantasy for the way it connects to the mind's creativity and imagination as a colorful escape to distant lands of mystical beasts and fantastic quests where the hero really does save the day. As she's matured artistically, Matthynssens has found writing to be a comforting counterbalance to a world where beloved characters don't always get back up after they fall down.

Matthynssens currently lives in Rochester, Minnesota and has four beautiful children and four wonderful grandchildren.

Cheryl was diagnosised with cancer in July of 2014 and have been fighting Cancer since that time. She has been in surgical recovery or on chemotherapy ever since.

www.ingramcontent.com/pod-product-compliance
Lightning Source LLC
Chambersburg PA
CBHW030356280726

48655CB00019B/2304